MASTER YOUR EMOTIONS FOR PREGNANT WOMEN

A practical guide to navigate and overcome negativity and better management of your feelings for pregnant women.

Dr. Marnie J. Saulter

All rights reserved. No part of this book may be reproduced or used in any manner without the written permission of the copyright owner except for the use of quotation in a book review.

Copyright © Dr. Marnie J. Saulter 2023

Table of contents

Introduction..**5**

The Significance of Emotions During Pregnancy..... 5

Setting Goals for Emotional Wellness...................... 6

Chapter 1: Understanding Pregnancy Emotions.....15

Introduction to Common Emotions......................... 15

Emotional Impact...20

Chapter 2: Managing Stress and Anxiety.................29

Recognizing Stress Triggers...................................29

Stress Reduction Techniques.................................. 31

Breathing Exercises and Relaxation.......................32

Chapter 3: Coping with Mood Swings......................33

Dealing with Hormonal Fluctuations......................33

Strategies for Balancing Mood................................35

Chapter 4: Partner and Family Support....................41

Communicating with Your Partner.......................... 41

Involving Your Family in Your Emotional Well-being...
43

Chapter 5: Self-Care During Pregnancy...................45

The Importance of Self-Care................................... 45

Practical Self-Care Tips.. 47

Chapter 6: Building a Support System.....................49

Finding Pregnancy Support Groups........................ 49

Seeking Professional Help When Needed..............51

Chapter 7: Preparing for Labor and Birth................ 53

Managing Fears and Anxieties............................... 53

Developing a Birth Plan..54
Chapter 8: Postpartum Emotional Wellness............59
The Emotional Rollercoaster After Birth................. 59
Coping with Postpartum Depression...................... 60
Chapter 9: Embracing Motherhood......................... 63
Adjusting to Life with a Newborn........................... 63
Balancing Motherhood and Self.............................64
Conclusion:...69
Reflection and Future Emotional Well-being.......... 70
Resources and Additional Reading...................... 71
<u>30- Days journal for you</u>

Introduction

Emotions During Pregnancy: Your Journey Begins

During pregnancy, you start on a unique and changing journey, one that extends beyond the physical changes in your body. It's a journey packed with a range of emotions, and how you traverse this emotional landscape may profoundly affect both your well-being and the health of your developing kid.

The Significance of Emotions During Pregnancy

Pregnancy is not simply about bodily changes; it's a deep emotional event. Your mental condition may impact your whole pregnancy experience, your baby's growth, and even your preparedness for parenting.

When you're pleased, your body produces chemicals that not only enhance your mood but also have a favorable influence on your kid. In contrast, worry and anxiety may lead to the production of stress hormones, which may impact your baby's growth and your personal well-being.

By understanding and controlling your emotions, you may create a more pleasant and supportive environment for your infant. Your mental well-being is not simply a personal affair; it's a gift you provide to your kid.

Setting Goals for Emotional Wellness

As you begin this path, consider creating emotional health objectives. These objectives may act as a compass, leading you through the many emotional states you'll experience throughout pregnancy. Here's a short activity to get you started:

Reflect on Your feelings: Take time to reflect about the feelings you've had since discovering your pregnancy. These could include delight, enthusiasm, anxiousness, or even terror. It's entirely natural to feel a combination of emotions.

Identify Your Emotional Priorities: What feelings would you prefer to experience more throughout your pregnancy? Perhaps you wish to nurture greater pleasure, relaxation, or thankfulness.

Create a List of Emotional Goals: Write down the exact feelings you wish to concentrate on throughout your pregnancy. For example, "I want to feel joy and gratitude throughout my pregnancy."

Review and Adjust: Revisit your emotional objectives frequently. As you go during your pregnancy, your emotional priorities may vary. Be open to altering your objectives to line with your developing requirements.

Your emotional experience throughout pregnancy is unique, and your emotional health objectives should match your own aspirations and requirements. This book is meant to help you reach your objectives, giving guidance, practical advice, and professional insights to assist you at every stage. So, let's go on this adventure together, with the objective of conquering your emotions for a better, healthier pregnancy.

Story of Sarah: A Pregnant Mother's Journey
Meet Sarah, a first-time mom-to-be. The instant the two pink lines emerged on the pregnancy test, her emotions started to whirlwind. Excitement, excitement, and expectation were at the forefront, but so were dread and uncertainty.

The First Trimester: Hopes and Fears
During the first trimester, Sarah's emotions were a rollercoaster. The thrill of becoming a mother was matched with worry for her baby's health.

Every pain or agony left her with a gnawing uncertainty. What if things went wrong? How could she safeguard this small life developing within her?

She also felt the weight of social expectations. Would she be a good mother? Could she combine her work and family? Would she have enough support? These were questions that kept her up at night, adding to the weariness of the first trimester.

The Second Trimester: A Ray of Sunshine

The second trimester brought a ray of light to Sarah's journey. Her morning sickness had subsided, and she began feeling her baby's mild flutters. She shared the news with her family and friends, which produced an outpouring of love and support.

Sarah's hopes started to soar. She began visualizing her baby's future, seeing a small hand wrapped around her finger, and dreaming of lullabies. The nursery was slowly taking form, and she was even contemplating baby names. It was a moment of optimism and aspirations.

The Third Trimester: Navigating Challenges

As Sarah neared her third trimester, additional obstacles developed. Her expanding tummy made regular duties a little more complex. She endured back discomfort, restless nights, and edema. The upcoming labor and delivery filled her with both excitement and fear. What would it be like? Would she be able to take the pain? Balancing work, doctor's visits, and the rising physical pain was tough. The financial ramifications of maternity leave weighed on her, too. Her emotions bounced from times of intense delight to periods of worry.

Throughout the Journey: Emotional Evolution

As Sarah advanced through her pregnancy, she learned to handle her emotions. She learnt that it's natural to experience a broad variety of emotions, and she found peace in connecting with other pregnant women who had similar fears.

Sarah came to embrace the notion of having emotional goals, realizing that she could strive for pleasure and relaxation while addressing her concerns and anxieties. With the support of her spouse, family, and a trusted healthcare team, she recognized that she wasn't alone on her path.

Sarah's emotional well-being developed, and she found the significance of self-care, stress management, and developing a support system. She learnt to enjoy the lovely moments of pregnancy and tackle the trials with bravery and tenacity.

Sarah's story is a tribute to the emotional complexity of pregnancy and the transforming power of knowing, controlling, and conquering your emotions throughout this magnificent journey. Throughout this book, we'll follow Sarah's adventures as she continues to manage her emotions and prepare for the birth of her little one.

Expert Insight: Dr. Emily Martinez

Dr. Emily Martinez is a highly recognized psychologist who has devoted her career to the issue of prenatal mental health. Her experience in the mental well-being of pregnant women and new moms has helped many people negotiate the sometimes challenging path of pregnancy and parenting.

Dr. Martinez underlines the vital significance that emotional control plays throughout pregnancy. She observes that pregnancy is not merely a medical process but a very emotional one. Every thought, sensation, and emotion a woman experiences may have a tremendous influence on her well-being and that of her kid.

"Pregnancy is a time of immense emotional intensity," explains Dr. Martinez. "Expectant moms experience a broad variety of emotions, from pleasure to dread and all in between.

Recognizing and regulating these emotions is crucial to a good pregnancy."

Dr. Martinez adds that the first stage is admitting your feelings, whether they're happy or bad. It's normal to experience a variety of emotions, and each one has its place in this changing path. Understanding and embracing your emotions is vital.

She also underlines the need of detecting indicators of mental strain. Sometimes, the strains of life, along with the hormonal changes of pregnancy, may lead to emotional issues. Dr. Martinez gives tips on spotting these indications and when to seek treatment.

"Never hesitate to reach out to a healthcare professional or therapist if you're struggling," she says. "Your emotional well-being is not just a personal matter; it's a vital component of your baby's development."

Dr. Martinez further notes that good emotions, including pleasure and relaxation, have a physical influence on the growing infant. When a woman feels pleasure and joy, her body produces hormones that help encourage a healthy pregnancy.

"Pregnant women should aim to create a nurturing environment for their babies," she recommends. "By managing emotions, practicing self-care, and seeking support, they can set the stage for a happier, healthier pregnancy."

Dr. Martinez's insights and counsel, helping you understand the importance of your emotions throughout pregnancy and providing you with useful methods to manage them for the benefit of both you and your baby.

Chapter 1: Understanding Pregnancy Emotions

Common Emotions During Pregnancy

Pregnancy is an amazing and transforming experience, and it's not unexpected that it comes with a flow of emotions. These feelings are as different as the colors of the rainbow, and each shade adds to the magnificent mosaic of your pregnant experience.

Introduction to Common Emotions

Excitement, delight, worry, fear, happiness, and uncertainty—it's totally natural to feel a tornado of emotions throughout pregnancy. Think of these feelings as the paint on the painting of your pregnant adventure. Each one adds depth, complexity, and richness to your unique tale.

Fear and Anxiety

Let's accept something essential: dread and worry are typical companions on the way to parenthood. It's totally natural to face moments of worry and anxiety as you navigate the undiscovered seas of pregnancy. Here are some of the frequent worries and anxieties pregnant women often face:

Fear of Labor: The idea of delivery may be scary. Many women worry about the pain, the uncertainty, and the unpredictability of the birth experience. It's acceptable to have these anxieties, and we'll examine strategies to handle them.

Changes in Lifestyle: Pregnancy brings considerable changes to your life. You could be anxious about how your relationships, job, and personal life will be impacted. These worries are genuine, and we'll give help on handling these changes.

Health of the kid: One of the most significant fears throughout pregnancy is the well-being of the kid. Will they be healthy? Is everything going as it should? It's typical to have these worries, and we'll cover ways to monitor and handle them.

Recognizing that fear and anxiety are part of the journey is the first step in handling them properly. It's crucial to recognize that you're not alone in feeling these emotions. In reality, they link you to many other pregnant women who have traveled this route before you.

Remember, it's good to have a variety of emotions; they are a part of your unique narrative.

Hormonal Fluctuations

One of the most astonishing parts of pregnancy is the delicate ballet of hormones that takes place inside your body. These hormone alterations are not only about bodily modifications; they play a crucial part in your emotional journey.

To further grasp this, let's take a basic look at the major hormones at play:

Human Chorionic Gonadotropin (hCG): This hormone is one of the early indications of pregnancy. It helps maintain the corpus luteum, which, in turn, generates progesterone. Early on, increased hCG levels might contribute to heightened emotions and possibly even morning sickness.

Progesterone: Often termed the "relaxing hormone," progesterone helps maintain the uterine lining and nourishes the growing fetus. However, it may also contribute to symptoms of weariness and mood changes.

Estrogen: This hormone swells throughout pregnancy and plays a crucial function in fetal growth. While it contributes to the "pregnancy glow" and a feeling of well-being for many, it may also produce emotional sensitivity and even episodes of weepiness.

Oxytocin: Known as the "love hormone," oxytocin is vital for birth and nursing. However, during pregnancy, it may promote emotions of connection and bonding, but it can also contribute to greater emotional sensitivity.

These hormone variations might be responsible for the emotional rollercoaster that some pregnant women experience. It's totally natural to swing from feeling ecstatic and passionately in love with your developing kid one minute to being gripped by tears and fear the next. The important thing is to recognize that these hormone swings are a normal part of the journey, and they impact each woman differently.

Emotional Impact

Now, let's discuss how these hormonal shifts might affect your mental state. Think of these hormones as the unseen strings that tug your emotional puppets. They can:

Amplify Emotional Sensitivity: Pregnancy hormones often intensify your emotional reactions. Small pleasures may seem more deep, yet tiny anxieties may build into enormous issues.

Cause Mood Swings: The variations in hormone levels might create mood swings, causing you to feel ecstatic one minute and despairing the next.

Increase weariness: Hormonal fluctuations may also add to weariness, which can further damage your emotional well-being.

Throughout this book, you'll hear from other pregnant women who've experienced emotional swings due to hormone imbalances. Sarah, our pregnant mother, will relate her experience, including times of hormonal-induced delight and those of vulnerability. These tales can help you recognize that you're not alone and that what you're experiencing is a typical aspect of the pregnant experience.

Understanding the significance of hormones in your emotional journey is a key first step in managing your emotions throughout pregnancy. It's crucial to remember that these oscillations are totally natural, and they are part of the lovely symphony that accompanies the birth of new life.

As Sarah's pregnant adventure proceeded, she learned directly how her body's hormonal symphony affected her emotional journey. It was a rollercoaster of ups and downs, sometimes within the same day.

The Hormonal Highs:
In the second trimester, Sarah started to feel the impact of rising hormones, which offered times of tremendous excitement. Her first ultrasound, when she saw her baby's tiny, fluttering heart, was a highlight. The flow of oxytocin at that time left her gushing with love and a tremendous connection to her developing kid.
Sarah felt herself smiling more frequently, full with optimism and joy about the tiny one she would soon hold in her arms. These highs carried with them a feeling of strength and purpose, as she came to embrace her position as a mother.

The Hormonal Lows:
However, Sarah also endured the typical hormonal lows. The increasing levels of progesterone, which relaxed her muscles and readied her body for the baby's birth, occasionally left her feeling tired and emotionally susceptible. Simple activities, like

tying her shoelaces or getting out of bed, looked like tremendous obstacles.

There were days when worry crept in. Fears about the coming birth, worry about her changing physique, and the uncertainty of parenting took their toll. Her emotions might swiftly flip from optimism to anxiety and back again.

Coping with the Emotional Rollercoaster:
Sarah learnt that it was vital to address her feelings. She communicated frankly with her spouse, family, and friends about her highs and lows. She learned that expressing her experiences not only lessened the emotional burden but also linked her with others who had traveled a similar route.

To combat the hormonal fluctuations, Sarah employed mindfulness practices, which helped her remain anchored in the present moment. She learnt that relaxation techniques and deep breathing might reduce periods of worry and overload.

Self-care became a lifeline. Sarah indulged herself with warm baths, calming music, and times of quiet thought. She recognized that self-compassion was crucial to navigate the emotional volatility of pregnancy.

As Sarah's tale progressed, she learned that recognizing the function of hormones in her emotional journey was the first step toward managing her emotions. The awareness that it was alright to experience both highs and lows helped her to embrace the entire gamut of her moods and approach each day with resilience and grace. Her path was far from complete, but she was acquiring the skills and insights required to face the future with confidence.

Expert Insight: Dr. Lisa Turner, OB-GYN

Dr. Lisa Turner is a highly renowned obstetrician-gynecologist with significant expertise in assisting pregnant women through the complications of pregnancy. Her comprehensive awareness of the physiological and emotional elements of pregnancy makes her a great resource for women looking to manage their emotions throughout this transforming journey.

The Science Behind Hormonal Changes During Pregnancy

Dr. Turner takes us on a tour into the extraordinary science of hormone changes throughout pregnancy. She adds that these changes are not ordinary fluctuations but a well planned symphony that prepares your body for the huge responsibility of nursing and delivering a kid.

"Pregnancy is a profound biological event," explains Dr. Turner. "Your body undergoes a series of intricate hormonal changes to support fetal growth and development."

She says that one of the important hormones, hCG (human chorionic gonadotropin), is generated by the placenta and plays a critical function in early pregnancy. It instructs the corpus luteum to continue making progesterone, which is crucial for maintaining the uterine lining and sustaining the developing baby. This hormonal change may lead to periods of happiness but may also contribute to weariness and mood swings.

Dr. Turner also underlines the importance of estrogen, which increases throughout pregnancy, encouraging the development of the baby's organs. This hormone is not only responsible for the "pregnancy glow" but may also contribute to emotional sensitivity.

"It's vital to note that these hormone shifts," Dr. Turner continues, "are not only about mood swings. They are crucial for the health and well-being of both mother and baby."

Guidance on Managing Emotional Fluctuations

Dr. Turner gives excellent advice on handling emotional changes throughout pregnancy. She advocates for self-awareness and self-compassion, urging pregnant moms to acknowledge their feelings without condemnation.

"Acknowledging your feelings is the first step," she recommends. "It's vital to realize that every woman's emotional path is unique. What's most crucial is that you develop appropriate strategies to deal with your feelings."

Dr. Turner advocates adopting mindfulness and relaxation practices to assist maintain emotional equilibrium. She says that self-care, including regular exercise, proper sleep, and a balanced diet, may go a long way in regulating emotional well-being.

"Remember that seeking support is a sign of strength, not weakness," she advises expecting moms. "Whether through a healthcare provider or a trusted friend, sharing your emotions can help you navigate the emotional ups and downs of pregnancy more effectively."

Dr. Turner's findings give a better knowledge of the science underlying hormone changes throughout pregnancy and provide a path for preserving emotional equilibrium. Her counsel acts as a source of empowerment for pregnant moms, allowing them to control their emotions throughout this incredible journey.

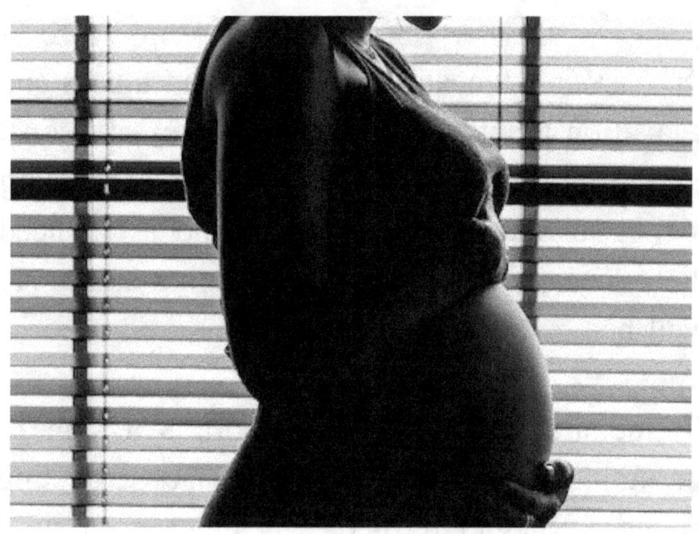

Chapter 2: Managing Stress and Anxiety

Pregnancy is a magnificent adventure filled with hope, expectation, and love, but it may also bring periods of tension and anxiety. As your body experiences physical changes, your mind navigates a plethora of emotions. In this chapter, we will discuss effective techniques to identify and manage the tension and anxiety that may be a part of this transforming process.

Recognizing Stress Triggers

Understanding what causes your stress is the first step toward controlling it. Stress causes may differ from one individual to another, but frequent sources of stress during pregnancy include:

Health Concerns: Worries about the baby's health or your personal well-being might be stressful. Understanding these problems and resolving them is key.

Financial Worries: Preparing for a new addition to the family typically comes with financial hardship. We'll examine solutions for handling this worry.

Work-Related Pressure: Balancing work and pregnancy may be tough. We'll discuss techniques to maintain a good work-life balance.

Relationship Dynamics: Changes in relationships, whether with a spouse, family, or friends, may lead to emotional stress.

The Unknown of Labor and delivery: The unknown of what labor and delivery will be like may contribute to severe anxiety.

We will take you through the process of detecting these stress triggers and understanding how they affect you. Self-awareness is the key to successful stress management.

Stress Reduction Techniques

Managing stress is vital for your mental well-being and the health of your kid. Here are some practical strategies to help minimize stress throughout your pregnancy:

Mindfulness & Meditation: These techniques may help you be present in the now and lessen worry about the future.

Exercise: Regular physical exercise may increase mood and decrease stress. We'll explore healthy workout alternatives for pregnant ladies.

Time Management: Learning to prioritize and manage your time wisely helps relieve the burden of a hectic schedule.

Journaling: Keeping a pregnant diary may give an outlet for your thoughts and feelings.

Breathing Exercises and Relaxation

Breathing exercises may be a lifesaver during periods of stress and worry. We'll offer easy strategies to quiet your mind and body, such as deep breathing and gradual muscle relaxation. These strategies will create pockets of peace throughout your day, delivering reprieve from the pressures of pregnancy.

By the conclusion of this chapter, you will have a toolset of ways to handle stress and anxiety efficiently. This information and these strategies will allow you to maintain emotional balance and find moments of serenity among the lovely turmoil of pregnancy.

Chapter 3: Coping with Mood Swings

Pregnancy is a beautiful journey filled with moments of excitement, anticipation, and love. Yet, it's also a period when mood fluctuations may rush in like a sudden thunderstorm. These emotional changes are natural, but recognizing and efficiently controlling them may dramatically improve your overall well-being. In this chapter, we will investigate the reasons for mood swings during pregnancy, present practical techniques to balance your mood, and share real-life insights to help you negotiate this emotional rollercoaster.

Dealing with Hormonal Fluctuations

Pregnancy is typically accompanied by a hormonal dance that might alter your emotions. Understanding the relationship between these hormonal changes and your mood swings is the first step in controlling them. Here's a short glance at the major hormones involved:

Progesterone: This hormone, crucial for supporting a healthy pregnancy, may occasionally contribute to symptoms of weariness and mood changes.

Estrogen: While responsible for the iconic "pregnancy glow," it may also heighten emotional sensitivity, often leading to mood swings.

Oxytocin: Known as the "love hormone," oxytocin stimulates connection and bonding but may also contribute to emotional volatility.

HCG (Human Chorionic Gonadotropin): Early in pregnancy, surges of this hormone may contribute to heightened emotions and even morning sickness.

Understanding that these hormones are causing your mood swings is liberating. It's a reminder that you're not alone, and that these emotional swings are a normal part of your particular pregnant experience.

Strategies for Balancing Mood

Balancing your mood throughout pregnancy is crucial for your emotional well-being. Here are some techniques to help you maintain a more steady emotional state:

Self-Care: Prioritize self-care habits like relaxation exercises, mindfulness, and treating yourself. These hobbies might give a breather from the maelstrom of emotions.

Lifestyle alterations: Make alterations to your regular routine to decrease stress. This might involve limiting your workload, obtaining appropriate rest, and ensuring you have a support structure in place.

Effective Communication: Open, honest communication with your spouse, friends, and healthcare provider is vital. Sharing your feelings and seeking assistance might help you manage more successfully with mood swings.

As Sarah's pregnancy proceeded, so did her emotional journey. The emotional intricacy of pregnancy became even more obvious as she dealt with mood swings that frequently arrived unexpectedly, like surprise guests at a party.

The Moments of Joy and Anticipation:

During the second trimester, Sarah had moments of incomparable delight and anticipation. The scan showed the gender of the baby, and the room erupted with laughter and tears of pleasure. She felt the baby's delicate movements, a calming presence that inspired a feeling of amazement and profound connection.

Sarah and her partner committed time to prepare for their baby's birth, constructing a pleasant nursery filled with soothing hues and careful care. These times were filled with optimism and enthusiasm, reminding her of the amazing trip she was on.

Navigating Emotional Turbulence:
Yet, Sarah also endured periods of emotional upheaval, typified by moments of heightened sensitivity, occasional irritation, and sometimes unexpected tears. These mood fluctuations might be prompted by apparently inconsequential things—perhaps a passionate commercial or a benign statement from a coworker.
The concerns and uncertainty of being a mother sometimes weighed heavy on her heart. Thoughts about the coming delivery, her capacity to care for a baby, and the changes in her body whirled in her head. These ideas occasionally lead to periods of self-doubt and emotional vulnerability.

Coping with Mood Swings:
Sarah was resolved to negotiate her emotional swings with grace and perseverance. She knew that these mood swings were part of the trip, just

as much as the joyous times. She started practicing mindfulness practices to be anchored in the present, which helped her control her emotional changes.

Her husband played a crucial role in her emotional journey, delivering constant support and understanding throughout the tough moments. Sarah took peace in knowing that her feelings, whether high or low, were welcomed and cherished by her loved ones.

The practice of self-care became an integral element of her regimen. She embraced relaxation techniques, spent time in nature, and decorated her house with calming music and smells. These self-care routines worked as a refuge of calm inside the unstable emotional terrain.

As Sarah's pregnancy proceeded, she discovered that controlling mood swings was not about eliminating them but about embracing the whole gamut of emotions. The experience was a voyage of self-discovery and emotional development, enabling her to prepare for the pleasures and hardships of parenthood with courage and perseverance.

With this guidance, you may discover emotional balance, promoting a more pleasant and stable emotional experience throughout this incredible trip.

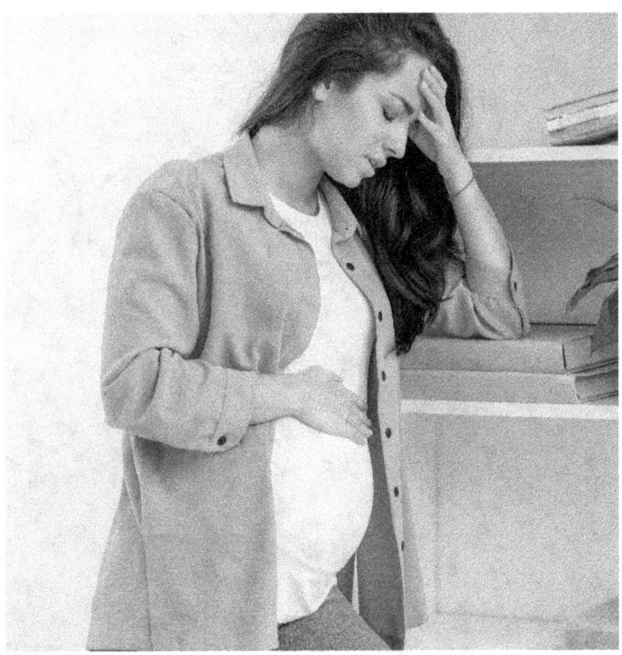

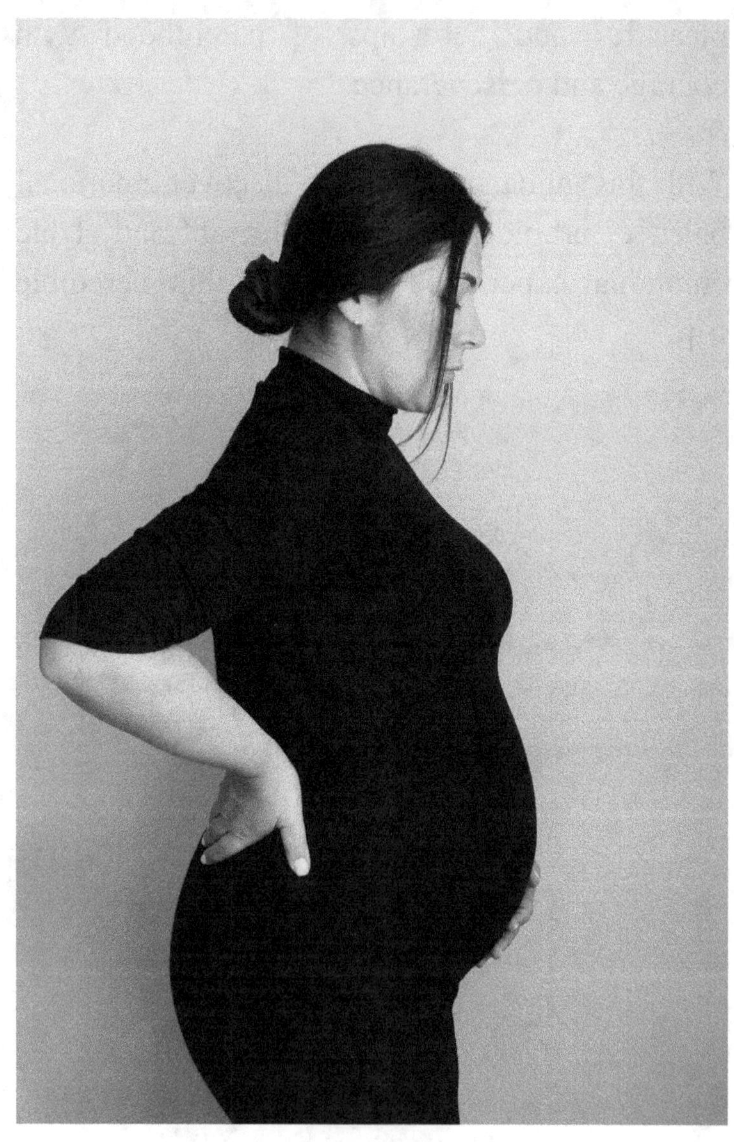

Chapter 4: Partner and Family Support

Pregnancy is a shared adventure, and the support of your spouse and family may be a precious source of strength and comfort during this transformational time. In this chapter, we will look into the value of efficient communication with your spouse and the role your family may play in supporting your emotional well-being.

Communicating with Your Partner

Your spouse is not merely a companion on your adventure; they are your co-pilot, your anchor in the storm, and your source of love and understanding. Effective communication with your spouse may dramatically improve your mental well-being throughout pregnancy.

The Importance of Open and Honest Communication:

Open and honest discussion is the cornerstone of a good collaboration. Sharing your feelings, fears, and pleasures is a wonderful approach to enhance your friendship. Your spouse may not entirely understand what you're going through, but by opening up, you bring them into your world, enabling them to be a source of support and comfort.

Expressing Your Needs:

Your lover is not a mind reader. Clearly stating your demands is vital. Whether it's a need for physical comfort, mental reassurance, or practical support, stating what you want may ease stress and provide a loving atmosphere for both you and your baby.

Involving Your Family in Your Emotional Well-being

The involvement of your family in your mental well-being throughout pregnancy is crucial. They are your foundation, your past, and your future. Here's how you may include your family in this amazing journey:

Seeking Assistance with Practical Matters:
Pregnancy may bring physical pain and limits. Your family may be a fantastic source of aid. Whether it's assisting with domestic tasks, running errands, or just giving a supporting shoulder, their efforts may lessen your burden.

Sharing Your Experiences:
Your family, particularly those women who have experienced pregnancy, may be a wealth of information and advice. Sharing your experiences with others and seeking their perspectives may generate a feeling of togetherness and connection.

Active Participation:
Encouraging your family's active engagement in your pregnancy journey helps establish a loving and caring culture. From attending doctor's visits to helping in newborn preparations, their presence may be a source of pleasure and connection.

Effective communication and their active engagement can not only improve your experience but also create a caring and supportive atmosphere as you prepare to welcome your little one.

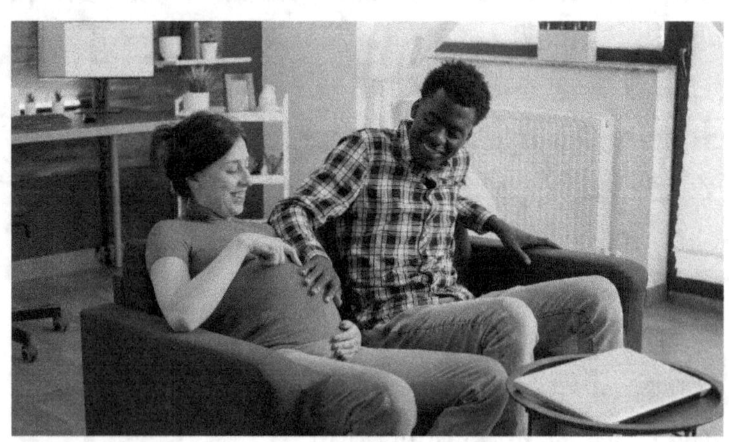

Chapter 5: Self-Care During Pregnancy

Pregnancy is an incredible time, but it can also be physically and emotionally stressful. In this chapter, we will discuss the crucial topic of self-care throughout pregnancy. We'll explain why self-care is vital, how it affects your mental well-being, and present you with a practical self-care toolbox customized to pregnant women.

The Importance of Self-Care

Self-care is not a luxury; it's a need, particularly during pregnancy. Taking care of oneself is not selfish but vital for your well-being and the health of your kid. Here's why self-care matters:

Nurturing Your Emotional Health:
Self-care is a valuable strategy for preserving emotional equilibrium. It enables you to manage stress, decrease anxiety, and produce a feeling of serenity amongst the emotional changes of pregnancy.

Promoting Physical Health:
Self-care is taking care of your physical well-being via healthy eating, exercise, and relaxation. A healthy physique may substantially affect your mental condition.

Creating a Positive Environment:
By emphasizing self-care, you create a caring and loving atmosphere for yourself and your kid. This favorable environment might improve your emotional well-being.

Practical Self-Care Tips

Self-care is not a one-size-fits-all idea. It incorporates a variety of procedures that may be adjusted to your individual requirements. Here are some practical self-care advice for pregnant women:

Relaxation Exercises: Incorporate relaxation methods like deep breathing, meditation, or awareness into your everyday routine.

Healthy Eating: A balanced diet rich in nutrients not only promotes your physical health but also adds to mental well-being.

Physical Activity: Engage in safe and moderate physical activities that enhance both physical and mental wellbeing.

Rest and Sleep: Ensure you obtain appropriate rest and sleep, which are crucial for emotional equilibrium.

Creative Outlets: Pursue creative pursuits that provide delight and relaxation, whether it's sketching, writing, or crafts.

Social Connections: Stay connected with friends and family who give emotional support and understanding.

These tactics will help you to nurture your mental health, maintain balance, and create a healthy environment for both you and your growing baby.

Chapter 6: Building a Support System

Pregnancy is a transforming experience that may be made more bearable and fulfilling with the correct support system in place. In this chapter, we'll cover the significance of creating a solid support network, including identifying pregnant support groups and obtaining professional aid when required.

Finding Pregnancy Support Groups

Pregnancy, with its mental and physical changes, may sometimes leave you feeling alone. Pregnancy support groups are a useful resource that may offer you with a feeling of community and understanding. Here's everything you need to know about them:

Benefits of Joining Support Groups:
Pregnancy support groups give a secure area to discuss experiences, worries, and pleasures.

Being part of a group of pregnant women may help normalize your emotional journey and create a feeling of connection.

How to Find Support Groups:
You may locate pregnancy support groups both in person and online. Your healthcare practitioner may offer suggestions, or you might seek on social media or pregnancy forums. Local community centers and hospitals typically organize support group meetings as well.

What to Expect from Support Groups:
Support groups may vary in format. Some are guided by experts, while others are peer-led. Expect frank talks, sharing of experiences, and practical advice. The emphasis is on emotional support, reassurance, and knowledge exchange.

Seeking Professional Help When Needed

Sometimes, the emotional problems of pregnancy may become overpowering, and that's when professional treatment might be needed. Here's everything you need to know:

When to Seek Professional Help:
If you feel that your emotional well-being is adversely impacted by anxiety, depression, or other mental health disorders, it's vital to get professional support. Additionally, if you're experiencing a high-risk pregnancy or difficulties, you may benefit from expert care.

Finding the Right Healthcare Provider or Counselor:
Your healthcare provider may be a great resource in connecting you with the correct specialists. Additionally, reaching out to a mental health counselor or therapist with expertise in prenatal care may give you the precise help you need.

What to Expect from Professional Support:
Professional aid may include therapy, counseling, or medication if required. The purpose is to assure your mental well-being and address any worries or difficulties you may be encountering throughout your pregnancy.

Building a solid support system is vital for preserving emotional balance and well-being throughout pregnancy. Whether via support groups or professional aid, broadening your network may give the understanding and resources you need as you continue on your particular path towards parenthood.

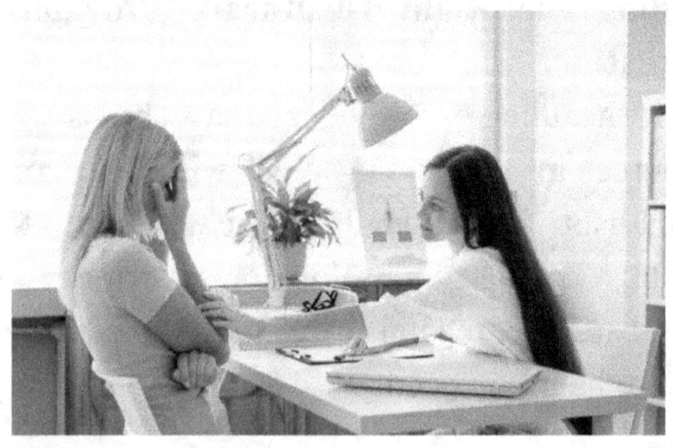

Chapter 7: Preparing for Labor and Birth

The journey of pregnancy is a lovely route that finally leads to one of the most momentous events of your life — the birth of your kid. In this chapter, we will discuss how to prepare for labor and delivery, addressing the management of worries and anxieties that might occur and the formulation of a birth plan that represents your particular goals.

Managing Fears and Anxieties

As you approach labor and delivery, it's typical to have concerns and anxiety. The prospect of the unknown might be scary, but you can negotiate this emotional terrain with grace. Here's how:

Understanding Common Fears and Anxieties: We'll address typical fears and anxieties associated with labor, such as dread of pain, concerns about complications, or anxiety about the delivering process. By recognizing these problems, you may begin to address and manage them effectively.

Strategies for Addressing Fears:
Facing your worries and concerns head-on is a powerful technique. We'll examine solutions to address these issues, including information, discussion with your healthcare physician, and relaxing techniques.

Support Systems:
Your support system, including your spouse and family, may play a key role in helping you manage your fears and anxieties. Open and honest contact with them may bring comfort and a feeling of security.

Developing a Birth Plan

A birth plan is your guide for the delivery experience you want. Creating one may empower you to make educated decisions and convey your preferences to your healthcare staff. Here's everything you need to know:

Components of a Birth Plan:

A birth plan is a personalized document outlining an individual's preferences for labor, delivery, and postpartum care. It typically includes personal information, healthcare provider details, and the chosen birthing environment. Preferences regarding pain management, labor interventions, and support people are key components. The plan often covers birthing choices, such as pushing preferences, episiotomy considerations, and newborn care, including immediate skin-to-skin contact and delayed cord clamping. Feeding choices (breastfeeding or formula) and postpartum care, including rooming-in and visiting preferences, may also be specified.

It's important to communicate potential scenarios and decisions in unexpected situations. Birth plans can express any unique requests or cultural traditions. While birth plans serve as a guide for medical professionals, they require flexibility as childbirth can be unpredictable. Discussing the plan with the healthcare provider is crucial to ensure alignment with medical needs and birthing facility policies. Overall, a birth plan is a tool that empowers expectant parents to advocate for their preferences during the birthing process, fostering a more personalized and comfortable experience while adhering to the highest standards of medical care and safety.

Flexibility and Communication:
In the context of pregnancy, flexibility and communication are essential. Pregnancy brings physical changes, emotional fluctuations, and numerous healthcare decisions. Flexibility helps expectant mothers adapt to bodily transformations and emotional variations while being open to adjustments in their prenatal journey. This includes embracing changes in plans, birth preferences, and healthcare decisions as needed.

Effective communication plays a vital role for pregnant women. It involves clear and open dialogue with healthcare providers to receive proper prenatal care and discuss any concerns. Communication with partners and support networks is essential for emotional support and ensuring others understand the woman's needs. A well-communicated birth plan helps ensure a smoother labor and delivery experience, aligning preferences with the medical team.

In sum, pregnant women benefit from maintaining flexibility to adapt to the dynamic nature of pregnancy and from nurturing open and effective communication with healthcare providers, partners, and support networks to create a supportive and informed environment throughout this transformative experience.

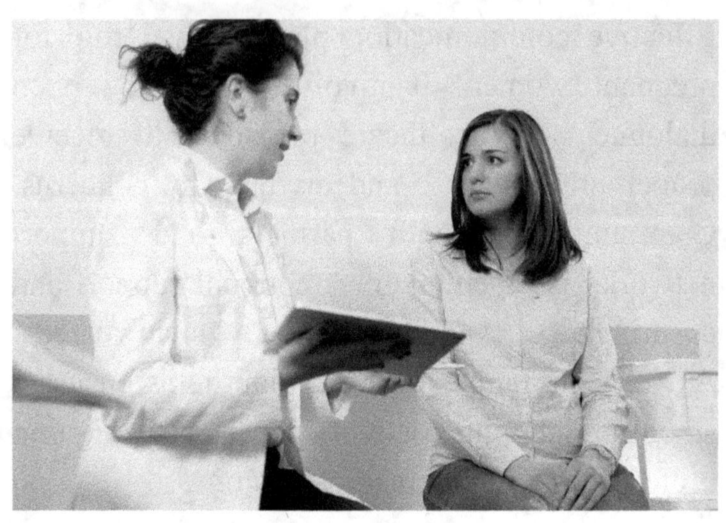

Chapter 8: Postpartum Emotional Wellness

The birth of your kid is a significant event, but it's vital to realize that your journey continues into the postpartum period. This chapter focuses on the emotional element of postpartum experiences, covering the emotional rollercoaster that may follow delivery and offers assistance on dealing with postpartum depression.

The Emotional Rollercoaster After Birth

After the birth of your kid, you're likely to feel a broad variety of emotions. The emotional rollercoaster might include moments of pleasure, love, and enormous satisfaction, but it may also contain tiredness, anger, and even melancholy. It's crucial to acknowledge that these emotional changes are part of the postpartum experience:

The Baby Blues: Many new moms endure what's generally known as the "baby blues." This entails bouts of feeling overwhelmed, weepy, or nervous. It's often a transitory period that may be ascribed to hormonal imbalances, lack of sleep, and the massive adjustment to parenthood.

Navigating the Emotional Complexity: Navigating these complicated emotions takes patience, self-compassion, and assistance. Lean on your support system, including your spouse, family, and friends. Open and honest communication might be your best ally at this time.

Coping with Postpartum Depression

While the baby blues are normal, some moms may have a more serious disorder known as postpartum depression. This is a significant mental health disorder that needs attention and care:

Signs and Symptoms: Postpartum depression is characterized by persistent emotions of melancholy, despair, and even a lack of interest in the infant. Other symptoms may include changes in diet and sleep habits, trouble connecting with the infant, and thoughts of self-harm or injuring the baby.

Seeking Help: Recognizing the signs and symptoms of postpartum depression is vital. If you feel you or someone you know is suffering postpartum depression, obtaining support from a healthcare physician or mental health expert is crucial. Postpartum depression is curable, and early intervention may make a major impact.

Strategies for Coping: Coping with postpartum depression includes a mix of professional help, medicine, and therapy. Additionally, support from your loved ones is crucial. Rely on your support network to assist you through this hard moment.

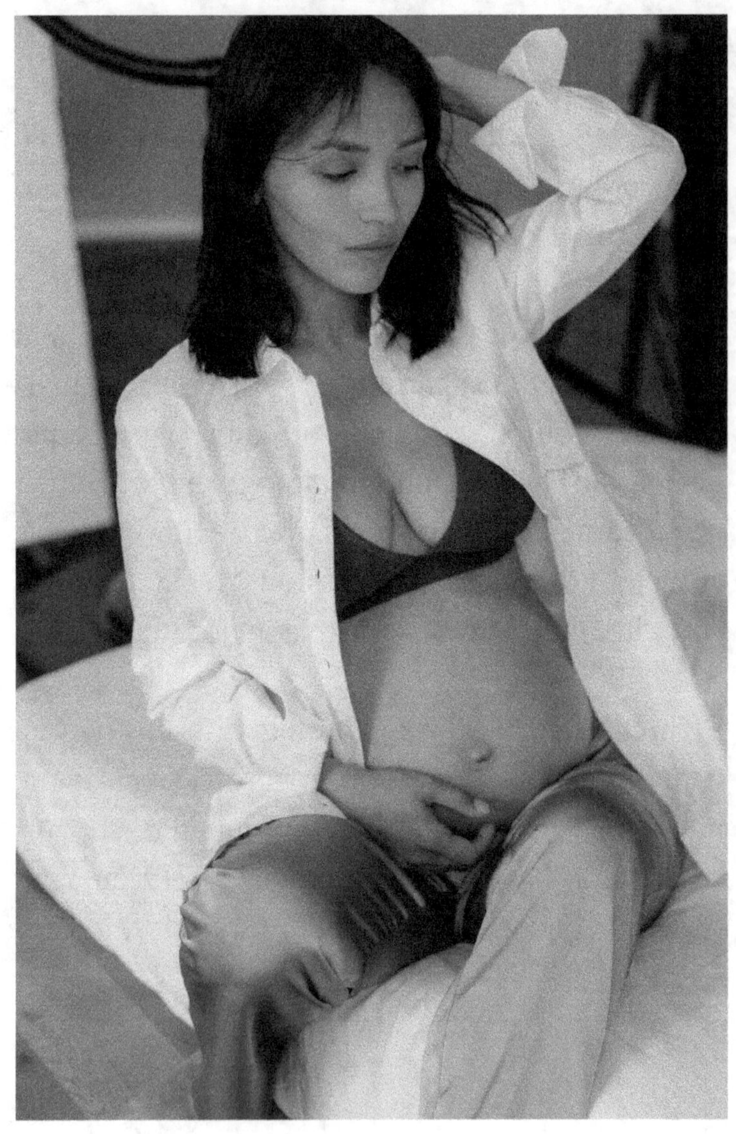

Chapter 9: Embracing Motherhood

Motherhood is a transforming and lifetime experience, and this last chapter is devoted to helping you accept your new position. We'll cover the changes and the skill of balance as you move into parenting.

Adjusting to Life with a Newborn

The birth of your kid is a huge life event, but it also represents the beginning of a big transition phase. Caring for a baby comes with its own set of difficulties and benefits, including:

Eating and Sleep Routines: Maintaining healthy eating and sleep routines is crucial for pregnant women and new mothers as they navigate the challenging yet rewarding phases of pregnancy and life with a newborn.

During pregnancy, a balanced diet is fundamental. Ensuring a well-rounded intake of nutrients is vital for both the mother's and baby's well-being. Frequent, smaller meals can help manage pregnancy-related discomfort, and staying hydrated is essential. Healthy snacks can provide sustained energy levels.

Sleep routines during pregnancy should focus on creating a comfortable sleep environment and following a consistent schedule. Relaxation techniques can alleviate discomfort and promote better sleep.

Adjusting to life with a newborn brings new challenges. Newborn feeding schedules may be irregular, especially with breastfeeding. A nutrient-rich diet remains important for both the mother's health and the quality of breast milk. Healthy snacks should be readily available.

Sleep routines post-birth can be fragmented due to the baby's unpredictable sleep patterns. Napping when the baby does can help recharge energy. Sharing nighttime duties with a partner can provide much-needed rest. Establishing a bedtime routine for the baby can aid in distinguishing day from night.

Flexibility is key in both phases. Self-care is a priority, and seeking support from family and friends is valuable. Personalized advice from healthcare providers on nutrition and sleep routines is highly recommended, as every pregnancy and newborn is unique. In the end, healthy routines enhance the well-being of both mother and child during these transformative stages of life.

Infant growth: understanding infant growth and adjusting to life with a newborn involves embracing the physical, cognitive, and emotional development of the child while being prepared for the practical and emotional adjustments required as new parents. Communication, support, and patience are key elements for a smooth transition into parenthood.

Balancing Motherhood and Self

While parenting is a crucial aspect of your life, it's essential to realize that you are more than simply a mother. Balancing parenthood with self is a difficult but vital skill. Here's how to accomplish it:

Self-Care: Taking care of oneself is not a luxury; it's a need. We'll discuss self-care strategies that may help you maintain your physical and mental well-being.

Maintaining own Interests: Nurturing your own interests and activities outside of parenthood may be gratifying. We'll address the significance of following your hobbies and keeping your distinct identity.

Nurturing connections: Motherhood should not separate you from your connections. We'll stress the value of keeping ties with your spouse, friends, and family, and how to manage these relationships with the demands of parenting.

Emotional Well-being: Emotional well-being is vital for pregnant women, and mastering their emotions is essential during this transformative period. It entails self-awareness, stress management, and open communication. Self-care, a strong support system, and education about pregnancy's emotional aspects are crucial. Accepting the range of emotions that come with pregnancy is a significant part of this process. By mastering their emotions, pregnant women can navigate the emotional complexities of pregnancy, reduce stress, and prepare for the arrival of their new baby with greater confidence and peace of mind.

Embracing parenthood entails cherishing your unique path while fostering your personal well-being and that of your tiny one.

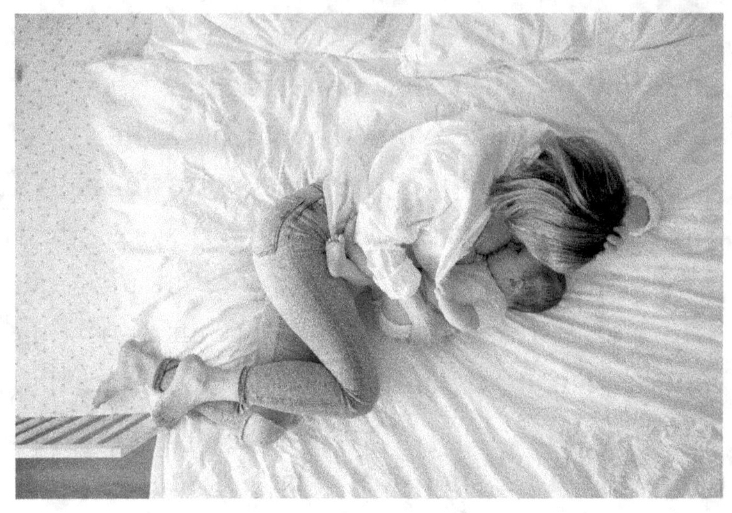

Conclusion:

Your experience through "Master Your Emotions for Pregnant Women" has been a fascinating one. Throughout this book, we've explored the emotional geography of pregnancy, from the first flutter of expectation to the momentous moments of labor and beyond. Your emotional well-being throughout this transitional moment is not just necessary; it's critical. Emotions define your experience, influence your health, and affect your baby's growth.

In this last chapter, we'll reflect on the emotional journey you've traveled and look forward to future emotional well-being. We'll also supply you with more resources and reading materials to further your investigation of this important issue.

Reflection and Future Emotional Well-being

Take time to reflect on your adventure. As you've read through this book, you've acquired insights about the usual emotions of pregnancy, the influence of hormone changes, and the tactics for controlling mood swings. You've followed Sarah's narrative and learnt about the importance of your support system. You're now equipped for the emotional terrain of postpartum and the skill of blending parenthood with self.

But remember, emotional well-being is a continuous journey. As you continue your journey into motherhood, think of the emotional skills you've learned here. Practice self-care, seek assistance when required, and remember that your mental health is as vital as your physical well-being.

Resources and Additional Reading

To further assist your mental well-being and broaden your knowledge, here are some more resources and reading materials:

"What to Expect When You're Expecting" by Heidi Murkoff and Sharon Mazel: A complete guide to pregnancy and the emotions that come with it.

"The Postpartum Husband: Practical Solutions for Living with Postpartum Depression" by Karen R. Kleiman: A resource for spouses to understand and assist postpartum emotional well-being.

"The Fourth Trimester: A Postpartum Guide to Healing Your Body, Balancing Your Emotions, and Restoring Your Vitality" by Kimberly Ann Johnson: A guide to handling the postpartum period emotionally and physically.

Online pregnancy forums and support groups: Connect with other expecting and new moms for shared experiences and support.

Local and online counseling services: Seek professional treatment if you're having emotional issues beyond what is common throughout pregnancy or after.

Remember, emotional well-being is a journey, and you have the skills and knowledge to navigate it effectively. Your emotions are a vital part of your unique pregnancy experience, and by controlling them, you're equipping yourself to accept the pleasures and trials of motherhood with courage, resilience, and a full heart.

30- Days journal for you

Pregnancy Emotional Journal

Date ______________

Weight ______________

Blood Pressure ______________

To Do

____
____
____
____

Cravings

____
____
____
____

Aversions

____
____
____
____

Thoughts and Feelings

____
____
____
____

Notes

____
____
____
____

Pregnancy Emotional Journal

Date ______________

Weight ______________

Blood Pressure ______________

To Do

____
____
____
____

Cravings

____
____
____
____

Aversions

____
____
____
____

Thoughts and Feelings

____
____
____
____

Notes

____
____
____

Pregnancy Emotional Journal

Date _______________

Weight _______________

Blood Pressure _______________

To Do

____
____
____
____
____

Cravings

____
____
____
____
____

Aversions

____
____
____
____

Thoughts and Feelings

____
____
____
____

Notes

____
____
____
____

Pregnancy Emotional Journal

Date ___________

Weight ___________

Blood Pressure ___________

To Do

____
____
____
____
____

Cravings

____
____
____

Aversions

____
____
____
____

Thoughts and Feelings

Notes

____
____
____
____

Pregnancy Emotional Journal

Date ______________

Weight ______________

Blood Pressure ______________

To Do

____
____
____
____

Cravings

____
____
____
____

Aversions

____
____
____
____

Thoughts and Feelings

____
____
____
____

Notes

____
____
____
____

Pregnancy Emotional Journal

Date _______________

Weight _______________

Blood Pressure _______________

To Do

____

____

____

____

Cravings

____

____

____

____

Aversions

____

____

____

____

Thoughts and Feelings

____

____

____

____

Notes

____

____

____

Pregnancy Emotional Journal

Date

Weight

Blood Pressure

To Do

Cravings

Aversions

Thoughts and Feelings

Notes

Pregnancy Emotional Journal

Date ___________

Weight ___________

Blood Pressure ___________

To Do

____
____
____
____
____

Cravings

____
____
____
____
____

Aversions

____
____
____
____
____

Thoughts and Feelings

____
____
____
____
____

Notes

____
____
____
____
____

Pregnancy Emotional Journal

Date

Weight

Blood Pressure

To Do

Cravings

Aversions

Thoughts and Feelings

Notes

Pregnancy Emotional Journal

Date _______________

Weight _______________

Blood Pressure _______________

To Do

Cravings

Aversions

Thoughts and Feelings

Notes

Pregnancy Emotional Journal

Date _______________

Weight _______________

Blood Pressure _______________

To Do

Cravings

Aversions

Thoughts and Feelings

Notes

Pregnancy Emotional Journal

Date _______________

Weight _______________

Blood Pressure _______________

To Do

____
____
____
____
____

Cravings

____
____
____
____
____

Aversions

____
____
____
____
____

Thoughts and Feelings

____
____
____
____
____

Notes

____
____
____
____

Pregnancy Emotional Journal

Date

Weight

Blood Pressure

To Do

Cravings

Aversions

Thoughts and Feelings

Notes

Pregnancy Emotional Journal

Date ___________

Weight ___________

Blood Pressure ___________

To Do

____
____
____
____
____

Cravings

____
____
____
____
____

Aversions

____
____
____
____

Thoughts and Feelings

____
____
____
____

Notes

____
____
____
____

Pregnancy Emotional Journal

Date ___________

Weight ___________

Blood Pressure ___________

To Do

Cravings

Aversions

Thoughts and Feelings

Notes

Pregnancy Emotional Journal

Date ___________

Weight ___________

Blood Pressure ___________

To Do

____
____
____
____
____

Cravings

____
____
____
____
____

Aversions

____
____
____
____

Thoughts and Feelings

____
____
____
____

Notes

____
____
____
____

Pregnancy Emotional Journal

Date ________________

Weight ________________

Blood Pressure ________________

To Do

____
____
____
____

Cravings

____
____
____
____

Aversions

____
____
____
____

Thoughts and Feelings

____
____
____
____

Notes

____
____
____
____

Pregnancy Emotional Journal

Date ______________

Weight ______________

Blood Pressure ______________

To Do

____
____
____
____

Cravings

____
____
____
____

Aversions

____
____
____
____

Thoughts and Feelings

____
____
____
____

Notes

____
____
____

Pregnancy Emotional Journal

Date

Weight

Blood Pressure

To Do

Cravings

Aversions

Thoughts and Feelings

Notes

Pregnancy Emotional Journal

Date ______________

Weight ______________

Blood Pressure ______________

To Do

____
____
____
____
____

Cravings

____
____
____
____
____

Aversions

____
____
____
____
____

Thoughts and Feelings

____
____
____
____
____

Notes

____
____
____
____

Pregnancy Emotional Journal

Date ___________

Weight ___________

Blood Pressure ___________

To Do

Cravings

Aversions

Thoughts and Feelings

Notes

Pregnancy Emotional Journal

Date ___________

Weight ___________

Blood Pressure ___________

To Do

Cravings

Aversions

Thoughts and Feelings

Notes

Pregnancy Emotional Journal

Date ___________

Weight ___________

Blood Pressure ___________

To Do

Cravings

Aversions

Thoughts and Feelings

Notes

Pregnancy Emotional Journal

Date ______________

Weight ______________

Blood Pressure ______________

To Do

____
____
____
____
____

Cravings

____
____
____
____
____

Aversions

____
____
____
____
____

Thoughts and Feelings

____
____
____
____
____

Notes

____
____
____

Pregnancy Emotional Journal

Date __________

Weight __________

Blood Pressure __________

To Do

____
____
____
____
____

Cravings

____
____
____
____
____

Aversions

____
____
____
____
____

Thoughts and Feelings

____
____
____
____
____

Notes

____
____
____
____

Pregnancy Emotional Journal

Date __________

Weight __________

Blood Pressure __________

To Do

____
____
____
____

Cravings

____
____
____
____

Aversions

____
____
____
____

Thoughts and Feelings

____
____
____
____

Notes

____
____
____
____

Pregnancy Emotional Journal

Date

Weight

Blood Pressure

To Do

Cravings

Aversions

Thoughts and Feelings

Notes

Pregnancy Emotional Journal

Date _______________

Weight _______________

Blood Pressure _______________

To Do

____
____
____
____

Cravings

____
____
____
____

Aversions

____
____
____
____

Thoughts and Feelings

____
____
____
____

Notes

____
____
____
____

Pregnancy Emotional Journal

Date ___________

Weight ___________

Blood Pressure ___________

To Do

____

____

____

____

Cravings

____

____

____

____

Aversions

____

____

____

____

Thoughts and Feelings

____

____

____

____

Notes

____

____

____

____

Pregnancy Emotional Journal

Date __________

Weight __________

Blood Pressure __________

To Do

____
____
____
____
____

Cravings

____
____
____
____
____

Aversions

____
____
____
____

Thoughts and Feelings

____
____
____
____

Notes

____
____
____

This book was created with the hope of providing you with insights, knowledge, and practical advice to navigate this remarkable journey with strength, resilience, and a full heart. We understand the challenges and joys that come with pregnancy and motherhood, and we're honored to be part of your support system.

Your feedback and reviews are invaluable. They not only help us improve but also guide other expectant mothers on their journey. We encourage you to share your thoughts, insights, and the impact this book had on your emotional well-being.

Thank you for trusting us as your companions on this transformative path. May your pregnancy and motherhood journey be filled with grace and joy, and may you master your emotions with confidence and resilience.

Thank you and have a happy journey ahead

www.ingramcontent.com/pod-product-compliance
Lightning Source LLC
Chambersburg PA
CBHW050737260726
48661CB00001B/284

9 798867 733070